Fatty Liver Low Carb Cookbook

35+ Curated and Tasty Low Carb Recipes to Manage Fatty Liver

mf

Disclaimer

By reading this disclaimer, you are accepting the terms of the disclaimer in full. If you disagree with this disclaimer, please do not read the guide.

All of the content within this guide is provided for informational and educational purposes only, and should not be accepted as independent medical or other professional advice. The author is not a doctor, physician, nurse, mental health provider, or registered nutritionist/dietician. Therefore, using and reading this guide does not establish any form of a physician-patient relationship.

Always consult with a physician or another qualified health provider with any issues or questions you might have regarding any sort of medical condition. Do not ever disregard any qualified professional medical advice or delay seeking that advice because of anything you have read in this guide. The information in this guide is not intended to be any sort of medical advice and should not be used in lieu of any medical advice by a licensed and qualified medical professional.

The information in this guide has been compiled from a variety of known sources. However, the author cannot attest to or guarantee the accuracy of each source and thus should not be held liable for any errors or omissions.

Table of Contents

Broccoli-Kale with Avocado Toppings Rice Bowl

Broccoli, Beans, and Squash Bowl

Roasted Broccoli and Salmon

Salmon and Crispy Kale (With Coconut)

Green Salad

Savory Chicken and Lentil Soup

Asparagus and Greens Salad with Tahini and Poppy Seed Dressing

Pine Nut Quinoa Bowl

Spinach Quiche

Broccoli Soup with Tumeric and Ginger

Avocado Chicken Lemon Salad

Asparagus with Garlic and Onions

Mixed Vegetable Roast with Lemon Zest

Conclusion

Introduction

Fatty liver is a condition that currently affects almost a third of the US population. This is mainly due to excessive alcohol consumption, unhealthy food choices, and sedentary lifestyles. Left unchecked, fatty liver can cause damage to the liver and lead to serious medical conditions such as liver fibrosis or scarring, and cirrhosis, which can be fatal.

As of this writing, there are no FDA-approved medications for the direct treatment of fatty liver. Fortunately, and if diagnosed early, this condition is easily reversible by making changes in the patient's diet and lifestyle.

Various studies have shown that a low-carb diet can help reverse the fatty liver disease or at least alleviate much of its symptoms.

This cookbook aims to provide a source of inspiration as to how one can get started cooking healthy, yet tasty low-carb meals that can help combat fatty liver disease.

A Brief Primer on the Fatty Liver Diet

One of the most effective approaches to fatty liver is through losing excess body fat. Health experts agree that 70% of weight loss is due to diet.

Although there are no FDA-approved drugs for the fatty liver yet, doctors agree that losing around 10% of the person's body weight is a good start, especially for patients who are obese.

NAFLD has been found most common for patients who live a sedentary lifestyle and those who consume mainly highly-processed foods.

Basic Components Of The Fatty liver Diet
A diet plan for people who have fatty liver should include the following:

- Lots of vegetables and fruits
- High-fiber foods like whole grains and legumes
- Reduced consumption of salt, sugar, refined carbohydrates, trans fat, and saturated fat
- No alcohol

The patient should undergo a reduced-calorie, low-fat diet to help in losing the excess weight.

Foods to Include in a Fatty liver Diet Plan

- Greens. In a study, broccoli has been found to be effective in helping prevent fat building in the livers of mice. Consuming more green vegetables like Brussels sprouts, spinach, and kale might also help with weight loss. There are a lot of vegetarian recipes that are full of flavor but low in calories.

- Coffee. Research has shown that those with fatty liver who also drink coffee are less susceptible to liver damage than those who don't. It's thought that the caffeine in this beverage reduces the levels of abnormal liver enzymes for those people that have high risks for liver diseases.

- Fish. Especially the fatty ones such as sardines, salmon, trout, and tuna, contain significant amounts of healthy omega-3 fatty acids. Omega-3 fatty acids have been found to help in improving fat levels in the liver and significantly reduce inflammation.

- Tofu. Soybeans have high protein content. Tofu is a soy product that has a high protein content but a very low fat amount. A study made on rats by the University of Illinois showed that soy protein reduces liver fat buildup.

- Walnuts. These contain high amounts of omega-3 fatty acids which, as previously discussed, have shown to be beneficial in improving liver function for patients diagnosed with fatty liver.

- Oatmeal. Carbohydrates consumed by patients with fatty liver should come from whole grains like oatmeal. Complex carbohydrates release a steady amount of energy and the fiber content satiates which is important in weight maintenance.

- Low-fat dairy. Whey protein might be able to help in protecting the liver from damage and this is important for those with fatty liver. Milk and other dairy products have high whey protein content but it's recommended for those with reduced fat content.

- Avocado. It might be high in fat content but these are the healthy ones. Research suggests that healthy fats and certain chemicals found in avocados can slow down liver damage. Avocados are also fiber-rich which helps in weight control.

- Olive oil. It's one of the healthiest and more readily available oils in the market. Olive oil is rich in omega-3 fatty acids and is much healthier when used for food preparation compared to shortening, butter, or margarine. Research shows that it can lower the number of liver enzymes and also help control weight.

- Sunflower seeds. The vitamin E content of the nutty-tasting sunflower seeds can protect the liver from damage due to its antioxidant properties.

- Green tea. From aiding with sleep to lowering cholesterol, green tea has shown many medical and health benefits. Initial studies show that green tea helps by interfering with fat absorption. It might also help with improving liver function and reducing fat storage in the organ.

- Garlic. It doesn't just add a lot of flavor and aroma to food but garlic powder supplements are also showing potential in the reduction of excess body weight for people with fatty liver.

Foods to Avoid
The following foods should be avoided or the consumption limited for patients with fatty liver. These contribute to increased blood sugar levels and weight gain which should be avoided when treating the disease.

- Alcohol. It's not only the major cause of the disease but also for other organ diseases.
- Fried food. These are soaked in fat and generally high in calories.
- Added sugar. Sugary foods such as cookies, candies, fruit juices, and soda should be avoided. High levels of sugar in the blood can increase liver fat buildup.
- Pasta, rice, and bread. Especially the white ones because the flour used has been highly processed. These can raise blood sugar levels. Opt for brown rice and whole wheat bread and pasta.

- Salt. Salt is linked to water retention and also causes fat buildup and high blood pressure but it's an essential ingredient of most foods. Limit consumption to no more than 1.5 grams per day.
- Red meat. Avoid deli meats and beef because these have high saturated fat content.

Sample Meal Plan 1

Meal	Menu
Breakfast	- Hot oatmeal (8 0z.), mixed with almond butter (2 tsp.) and sliced banana (1 pc.) - Coffee with skim or low-fat milk (1 cup)
Lunch	- Salad greens with olive oil and balsamic vinegar dressing - Grilled chicken, 3 oz. - Baked small potato - Cooked carrots or broccoli, 1 cup - Apple, 1 pc. - Milk, 1 glass
Snack	- Raw veggies with 2 tbsp. of hummus or sliced apples with 1 tbsp. peanut butter
Dinner	- Mixed-bean salad, small - Grilled salmon, 3 0z. - Cooked broccoli, 1 cup - Whole-gráin roll, 1 pc - Mixed berries, 1 cup - Milk, 1 glass

Sample Meal Plan 2

Meal	Menu
Breakfast	- High-fiber cereal with low-fat milk or multigrain bread (2 slices) with tomato / baked beans / peanut butter / mushrooms / cottage cheese - Fruit, 1 pc. - Water
Morning Tea	- Fruit (1 pc) / Greek yogurt (100 – 200 g) / oatmeal biscuits (2 pcs.) / fruit bread (1 thin slice) / grainy crackers with tomato and cottage cheese (2 pcs.) / raw nuts (5 to 6 pcs.)
Lunch	- 1 wrap / 1 bread roll / multigrain bread (2 slices) - Green salad with low fat cheese / chicken / salmon / tuna - Water
Afternoon Tea	- Fruit (1 pc) / Greek yogurt (100 – 200 g) / oatmeal biscuits (2 pcs.) / fruit bread (1 thin slice) / grainy crackers with tomato and cottage cheese (2 pcs.) / raw nuts (5 to 6 pcs.)
Dinner	- 120 g lean chicken / eggs / chicken

	/ legumes - Vegetables (zucchini / spinach / peas / cauliflower / carrots / cabbage / broccoli / beans - Whole wheat pasta (1 cup) / Brown rice (2/3cup) / sweet potato (1/2 cup) / medium potato (1 pc.) - Water

Grilled Chicken Breast

Ingredients:
- 4 pcs. skinless, boneless, chicken breasts
- 1 tbsp. sugar
- 1 tsp. garlic powder
- 2 tbsp. Italian seasoning
- 1 tbsp. pepper
- 1 tbsp. salt
- 2 tbsp. lemon juice
- 3 tbsp. Worcestershire sauce
- 2 tbsp. dijon mustard
- 1/4 cup cider vinegar
- 1/3 cup olive oil

Instructions:
1. Combine all of the ingredients in a Ziploc bag or large bowl. Massage or toss until well combined.
2. Marinade the chicken breasts for at least 30 minutes. You can also refrigerate for up to 4 hours.
3. Preheat the grill to medium to medium-high heat.
4. Place marinated chicken breasts on the grill and cook for 7 to 8 minutes.
5. Flip them over and cook for another 7 to 8 minutes. The internal temperature of the chicken should be 165 degrees when checked with a meat thermometer.
6. Take the chicken off the grill and place it on a serving plate.
7. Allow resting for 3 to 5 minutes before slicing and serving.

Mixed Bean Salad

Ingredients:
- 400 g. tin can mixed bean salad, drained and rinsed
- 2 stalks spring onions, finely chopped
- 2 sticks celery, thinly sliced
- 1 pc. large tomato, deseeded and finely diced
- salt
- freshly ground black pepper

For the dressing:
- 3 tbsp. olive oil
- 1 tbsp. white wine vinegar
- 1 tsp. sugar
- 2 tsp. Dijon mustard
- 1 tbsp. fresh tarragon, chopped
- 1 tbsp. fresh parsley, chopped

Instructions:
1. Put mixed beans, spring onions, celery, and tomato in a salad bowl.
2. Add salt and pepper to taste. Mix well.
3. In a separate bowl, mix ingredients for the dressing until well combined.
4. Pour the dressing on the salad and toss well.
5. Serve immediately.

Green Smoothie

Ingredients:

- 6 dandelion greens, chopped
- 4 kale leaves, stems removed, chopped
- 1 Meyer or organic lemon, peeled and sliced into chunks
- 1 Fuji apple, cut into chunks
- 2 cups filtered water
- Optional: 1 small banana, peeled and sliced
- Optional: 1 tsp. grated ginger

Instructions:
1. Place all ingredients into a blender
2. Blend on high speed for 1-2 minutes
3. Add more water if necessary.
4. Serve and enjoy.

Detox Juice

Ingredients:
- 1 beet, scrubbed
- 1 apple
- 1 lemon, peeled
- 1 cucumber, peeled
- one handful dandelion greens, washed

Instruction:

Juice   everything   and   stir   well.

Lentil Soup

Ingredients:

- 1 tbsp. vegetable oil
- 1 cup onion, diced
- 1/2 cup carrot, diced
- 1/2 cup celery, diced
- 4 cups vegetable or chicken broth
- 1 cup dried red lentils, well rinsed
- 1/4 tsp dried thyme
- 1/2 cup fresh flat-leaf parsley, chopped
- salt and pepper, to taste

Instructions:

1. Sauté carrot, celery, and onion in a large saucepan over medium heat. Do so until they are soft.
2. Pour in the broth, with lentils and thyme and wait for it to boil.
3. Lower the heat. Cover and leave to simmer until lentils are soft, about 20 minutes.
4. Transfer soup into a blender.
5. Set the blender on high. Purée the soup until it's creamy.
6. If it's too thick, pour in a cup of water.
7. Add salt and pepper, to taste.
8. Return to the saucepan to reheat if necessary.
9. Ladle into bowls and garnish with parsley.
10. Serve and enjoy while hot.

Roasted Veggies

Ingredients:
- 1/2 lb. turnips
- 1/2 lb. carrots
- 1/2 lb. parsnips
- 2 shallots, peeled
- 1/4 tsp. ground black pepper
- 1 tbsps. extra-virgin olive oil
- 6 cloves garlic
- 3/4 tsp. kosher salt
- 2 tbsp. fresh rosemary needles

Instructions:
1. First, cut vegetables into bite-sized pieces.
2. Set the oven to 400°F.
3. Mix all the ingredients in a baking dish.
4. Roast the vegetables for 25 minutes until brown and tender.
5. Toss and roast again for 20- 25 minutes.
6. Serve and enjoy while hot.

Healthy Green Smoothie

Ingredients:
- 1 cup fresh spinach
- 1/2 tsp. mint extract or to taste
- Optional: 1/4 tsp. peppermint liquid Stevia

Instructions:
1. Gather the ingredients.
2. Add them to a high-powered blender.
3. Turn on the blender.
4. Add them to the glass and freeze for 5 minutes.
5. Serve and enjoy.

Chicken Masala Crockpot Style

Ingredients:

- 6 boneless skinless chicken breasts, halved lengthwise
- 2 cloves of minced garlic
- 2 tbsp. extra virgin olive oil
- 1 tsp. salt
- 1 tsp. pepper
- 2 cups Marsala wine or chicken broth
- 1 cup of cold water
- 1/2 cup arrowroot powder
- 16 oz. sliced baby Portobello mushrooms
- 3 tbsp. fresh parsley, chopped

Instructions:

1. Grease the slow cooker. Add garlic and oil.
2. Season chicken with salt and pepper on each side and lay in the crockpot.
3. Pour wine over the chicken and cover the crockpot.
4. Cook on high for 3 hours.
5. Mix water with arrowroot and stir until absorbed.
6. Remove chicken from the crockpot and keep warm.
7. Stir in arrowroot water mixture into the bottom of the crockpot. Add mushrooms.
8. Add back the chicken. Stir well to coat chicken with sauce and mushrooms.
9. Cover and cook for an additional hour.

10. Serve with a sprinkle of chopped fresh parsley.

Balsamic-Glazed Chicken Thighs

Ingredients:

- 1 tsp. garlic powder
- 1 tsp. dried basil
- 1/2 tsp. salt
- 1/2 tsp. pepper
- 2 tsp. dehydrated onion
- 4 garlic cloves, minced
- 1 tbsp. extra-virgin olive oil
- 1/4 cup balsamic vinegar
- 8 chicken thighs, boneless and skinless
- fresh chopped parsley, for garnish

Instructions:

1. Add the spices together in a dish and put this on the chicken
2. Pour oil on the crockpot and add garlic.
3. Pour in half of the balsamic vinegar.
4. Put the chicken on the top and then add more vinegar.
5. Cover and cook on high for 3 hours.
6. Sprinkle fresh parsley

Chicken Breasts (Baked)

Ingredients:

For the chicken breast:

- 4 chicken breasts, boneless and skinless
- 1 tbsp. olive oil
- 3 and a half cups of water

For the chicken seasoning blend:

- 1/4 tsp. salt and pepper to taste
- 1/2 tsp. garlic powder
- 1/8 tsp. pepper
- 1/2 tsp. rosemary
- 1/2 tsp. onion powder
- 1/2 tsp. dried thyme
- 1/3 tsp. paprika
- 1/3 tsp. parsley, dried or fresh, chopped, for garnish

Instructions:

1. Preheat the oven to 425°F.
2. Combine water and salt in a large bowl.
3. Add the chicken breasts. Leave 25 minutes
4. In a separate container, combine the dry ingredients of the seasoning blend with a fork.
5. Pour out the water and rinse the chicken until it's dry
6. Rub oil over the chicken and place into a dish that can be used for baking

7. Evenly apply the seasoning blend over the chicken on all sides.
8. Place in the oven to cook for 25 minutes.
9. Make sure to keep an eye on the breasts, as each piece may cook faster than the rest.
10. Broil the chicken until the top parts are golden.
11. Transfer to a serving plate to rest for 10 minutes before cutting.
12. Garnish with parsley upon serving.

Baked Salmon

Ingredients:

- 2 salmon fillets
- 6 cups of fresh spinach
- 2 tsp. coconut oil
- 1 tsp. coconut oil
- 1/4 tsp. garlic powder
- 1/4 tsp. turmeric
- 3 large cloves of garlic
- lemon juice
- salt and pepper, to taste

Instructions:

1. Preheat the oven to 400°F.
2. Line a baking dish with parchment paper.
3. Marinate salmon fillets in lemon juice, coconut oil, garlic powder, turmeric, salt, and pepper.
4. Let it sit for a few minutes. This may also be done the night before to help the juices and flavor get into the salmon.
5. Once the oven is ready, bake salmon for 15 minutes.
6. Cook some of the garlic in a pan with coconut oil.
7. Add spinach and cook until ready. Season with salt and pepper to taste.
8. Take salmon out of the oven and put spinach beside it.

9. Serve   and   enjoy.

Spinach and Watercress Salad

Ingredients:

- 1 cup watercress, washed with stems removed
- 3 cups baby spinach, washed with stems removed
- 1 medium sliced avocado
- 1/4 cup avocado oil
- 1/8 cup lemon juice
- a pinch of salt

Instructions:

1. Pat dry the spinach and watercress. Remove the stem and separate the leaves.
2. On a large serving plate, combine the leaves of the watercress and the spinach.
3. Cut the avocado in half then remove the pit. Peel the skin off from each side.
4. Slice the avocados into thin strips. Set aside.
5. Prepare the dressing by combining avocado oil and lemon juice.
6. Arrange the avocado strips on top of the watercress and spinach.
7. Season with salt and pepper.
8. Drizzle with the dressing before serving.

Carrot and Cashew Soup

Ingredients:
- 1/4 cup cashews, chopped
- 3 cups carrots, peeled and chopped
- 4 cups water
- 1 large leaf or 2 small sage leaves
- Freshly ground black pepper, to taste
- 1/4 tsp. salt

Instructions:
1. In a large pot, place carrots, cashews, and sage.
2. Add water and bring to a boil.
3. Reduce to a simmer. Cook until the carrots are tender.
4. Place the carrot mixture in a high-speed blender and process until exceptionally smooth, about a minute.
5. Before serving, reheat the soup and stir in salt and pepper.
6. If the soup is too thick, add a few tablespoons of water.
7. Serve and enjoy while hot.

Cucumber with Fennel and Creamy Avocado Dressing

Ingredients:
- 2 cups sliced cucumber
- 1/2 medium avocado, peeled and pit discarded
- 1/4 tsp. and a dash salt
- freshly ground black pepper, to taste
- 2 tbsp. fresh lemon juice
- 1 large fennel, outer layer removed
- 1 tbsp. finely chopped chives

Instructions:
1. In a large bowl, combine cucumber and fennel.
2. Toss with 1/4 tsp. of salt and pepper. Set aside.
3. In a food processor, combine avocado and lemon juice. Process until smooth for about 20 seconds.
4. Add the avocado mixture to the cucumber mixture. Combine thoroughly.
5. Add chives and a dash of salt.
6. Serve and enjoy at once.

Cod Burger

Instructions:

- 1/3 cup cracked wheat
- 1-1/2 lb. cod
- 1 tsp. lemon juice
- Canola oil cooking spray
- 1-1/2 cups cooked white beans, dry or canned, no salt added, rinsed and drained
- 1/2 cup chopped parsley
- 1/2 tsp. salt
- Freshly ground black pepper, to taste
- 2 tsp. olive oil

Instructions:

1. Place cracked wheat in a bowl. Cover with 1/3 cup of boiling water. Let sit until water is absorbed, about 10 minutes.
2. Preheat the oven to 375°F.
3. Place cod on a baking dish, coat with lemon juice and vegetable oil cooking spray.
4. Cook until the fish starts to flake with the center still translucent, approximately 7 minutes.
5. Purée white beans in a blender or food processor.
6. Remove fish from the oven, let cool, and flake into a large bowl.
7. Add cracked wheat, beans, parsley, pepper, and salt. Hand mix everything.

8. Form into burger patties. This can make about four.

9. Over medium heat, coat a heavy-bottomed skillet with olive oil.

10. Fry burgers until all the sides are brown, about 4 minutes on one side.

Salmon Salad

Ingredients:

- 2 large fillets of wild salmon, either poached or grilled and then chilled
- 1 cup cherry tomatoes, halved
- 2 red onions, sliced
- 1 tbsp. balsamic vinegar
- 1 tbsp. capers
- 1 tbsp. fresh dill, finely chopped
- 1 tbsp. extra-virgin olive oil
- 1/4 tsp. pepper, freshly ground
- A pinch of salt

Instructions:

1. Remove skin and bones from the cooled salmon.
2. Break salmon into chunks, and place into a bowl.
3. Add tomatoes, red onion, and capers. Toss ingredients.
4. Combine balsamic vinegar, olive oil, and dill in a separate bowl.
5. Pour the mixture over salmon chunks. Toss again.
6. Sprinkle with salt and pepper to taste.
7. Chill salad for at least half an hour before serving.

Asian Zucchini Salad

Ingredients:

- 1 medium zucchini, sliced thinly into spirals
- 1/3 cup rice vinegar
- 3/4 cup avocado oil
- 1 cup sunflower seeds, shells removed
- 1 lb. cabbage, shredded
- 1 tsp. stevia drops
- 1 cup almonds, sliced

Instructions:

1. Cut the zucchini spirals into smaller parts. Set aside.
2. Put almonds, sunflower seeds, and cabbage in a large bowl. Combine the ingredients well.
3. Add zucchini to the mixture.
4. In a small bowl, mix vinegar, stevia, and oil using a whisk or fork.
5. Pour vinegar mixture all over the zucchini mixture. Toss well. Make sure everything is covered with the dressing.
6. Refrigerate for 2 hours before serving.

Garlic Broccoli Salad

Ingredients:

- 1 head broccoli, cut into florets
- 1 tsp. olive oil
- 1-1/2 tbsp. rice wine vinegar
- 1 tbsp. sesame oil
- 2 cloves garlic, minced
- 1 pinch cayenne pepper
- 3 tbsp. golden raisins

Instructions:

1. Fill water into a steamer. Bring into a boil.
2. Add broccoli. Cover. Steam until tender for about 3 minutes.
3. Rinse broccoli and set aside.
4. Heat olive oil in a skillet over medium heat.
5. Put in pine nuts. Stir fry for 1-2 minutes.
6. Remove from heat.
7. Whisk together rice vinegar, sesame oil, pepper, and garlic.
8. Transfer the broccoli, nuts, and raisins to the rice vinegar dressing.
9. Serve and enjoy.

Zucchini Frittata

Ingredients:
- 1-1/2 cups zucchini, chopped
- 1-1/2 cups red onion, sliced
- 2 tbsp. extra virgin olive oil
- 7 eggs, beaten
- 2/3 cup mozzarella balls
- 1/2 tbsp. salt
- 3 tbsp. tomatoes, chopped
- 1/4 tsp. ground pepper
- 1/4 cup basil, sliced

Instructions:
1. Heat the oil in a cast-iron skillet. Wait until it's reached medium heat.
2. Add the onions and zucchini. Stir until they become soft.
3. Whisk the eggs in a separate bowl. Mix in salt and pepper.
4. Pour the egg on the zucchini and onions. Cook the egg and top the frittata with cheese, tomatoes, and basil.
5. Cut the frittata into four.
6. Serve and enjoy.

Avocado Kale and Mango Smoothie

Ingredients:
- 1/2 cups ripe avocado
- 1-1/2 cups kale, chopped
- 1 cup mango pulp
- 1/2 cup ice cubes

Instructions:
1. Put all ingredients into the mixer and blend.
2. Pour into 3 individual glasses and serve.

Minestrone Soup

Ingredients:
- 3 large carrots, diced
- 2 large onions, chopped
- 2 cloves garlic, minced
- 2 cups celery, chopped
- 1 cup green beans, cut in half-inch pieces
- 1.5 cups kidney beans, dried
- 1 large bell pepper, diced
- 1 cup frozen peas
- 1 can tomatoes, diced
- 2 cups tomato sauce
- 2 tbsp. fresh basil or 1 tsp. dried basil
- 6 cups water

Instructions:
1. In a stockpot over medium heat, add in the water, onions, carrots, and celery.
2. As the water starts to bubble, add in the green beans, bell pepper, peas, and tomatoes.
3. Let it bubble for around 30 minutes.
4. Add water if necessary. The soup should be thick, similar to a stew, but not too thick.
5. After half an hour, add the tomato sauce, beans, basil, and salt to taste.
6. Let it stew for 5-10 additional minutes at that point including the garlic. Let it stew for 5 additional minutes.
7. Serve while hot.

Asparagus and Greens Salad with Tahini and Poppy Seed Dressing

Ingredients:

For the salad:

- 10 to 12 asparagus stalks, washed well and sliced into ribbons
- 5 radishes, washed well and sliced thinly
- 2 to 3 rainbow carrots, peeled and sliced thinly
- 1 handful wild spinach
- 1 small handful of microgreens, washed well
- 1 small handful of sunflower greens, washed well
- Optional: few pieces of chive blossoms

For the dressing:

- 2 tbsp. tahini
- 1 tbsp. poppy seeds
- 1 tbsp. extra-virgin olive oil
- Salt and pepper, to taste

Instructions:

1. For the dressing, whisk ingredients together in a small bowl.
2. In a separate bowl, toss salad ingredients in the mixture.
3. Drizzle dressing on salad upon serving.

Pine Nut Quinoa Bowl

Ingredients:
- 1 cup white quinoa, rinsed

Sauce:
- 1/3 cup olive oil
- 1-1/4 tbsp. agave nectar
- 2 tbsp. lemon juice
- 2 cups sun-dried tomatoes
- 1 cup soaking water from tomatoes
- 1/2 onion
- 2 large heirloom tomatoes, chopped
- A handful of fresh basil leaves
- 4 garlic cloves, crushed
- 1 tsp. sea salt
- 2 tsp. dried oregano
- 1/4 cup pine nuts
- A pinch of hot pepper flakes

Instructions:
1. Boil quinoa with 2 cups of water. Reduce heat and let it simmer, covered, for about 18 minutes until quinoa is tender and water is absorbed.
2. In a blender, combine olive oil, lemon juice, and agave nectar.
3. Add tomatoes, onions, garlic, basil, oregano, salt, and hot pepper flakes.
4. Blend until it's smooth (water optional)

Asian Medley Bowl

Ingredients:

- 2 cups quinoa, cooked
- 4 carrots, washed and trimmed
- 1 package of smoked tofu
- 1 tbsp. nutritional yeast
- 2 tbsp. coconut aminos
- 4 tbsp. sunflower sprouts
- 2 tbsp. fermented vegetables
- 1 cup shiitake mushrooms
- 1 avocado
- 2 tbsp. hemp seeds
- 2-3 beets, cooked
- coconut oil cooking spray

For the dressing:

- 2 tbsp. miso paste
- 1 tbsp. tahini
- 1 clove garlic, crushed
- 1 tbsp. olive oil
- 1/2 lime, juiced
- 3 tbsp. water

Instructions:

1. Spray coconut oil on the carrots and roast in the oven at 400°F for 30-40 minutes.
2. Set aside till you are ready to assemble the Buddha bowl.
3. Combine all of the dressing ingredients in a medium-size bowl. If the dressing appears lumpy, add more water.
4. To build the bowl, put the quinoa on the bottom and then arrange the vegetables on top, sprinkle the bowls with hemp seeds, and drizzle the dressing over top.
5. Serve and enjoy.

Broccoli-Kale with Avocado Toppings Rice Bowl

Ingredients:

- 1/2 avocado
- 2 cups kale
- 1 cup broccoli florets
- 1/2 cup cooked brown rice
- 1 tsp. plum vinegar
- 2 tsp. tamari
- sea salt, to taste

Instructions:

1. In a small pot, simmer broccoli florets, and kale in about 3 tbsp. of water. Cook for 2 minutes.
2. Add tamari, vinegar, and cooked brown rice. Stir to combine.
3. Transfer pot contents into a medium-sized bowl and top with sliced avocado; sprinkle a dash of sea salt to taste.
4. Serve immediately.

Broccoli, Beans, and Squash Bowl

Ingredients:

- 1/2 cup brown rice
- 3 cup chard, roughly chopped
- 1 cup squash, diced
- 1 cup broccoli florets
- 1 cup black beans, rinsed and drained thoroughly
- 1 oz. kombu
- 1/2 cup sauerkraut, chopped

For the sauce:

- 2 tbsp. sesame tahini
- 2 tbsp. sodium tamari
- 1 clove garlic
- 1 tbsp. ginger
- 1 lime, juiced

Instructions:
1. Boil a cup of water. Add rice, allowing to boil.
2. Cover. Reduce heat and simmer for 40 minutes.
3. Remove from heat and allow to sit covered for an additional 10 minutes then fluff with a fork.
4. Place beans in a pot with kombu. Cover with water. Bring to a boil.

8. In a small bowl, combine the vinegar, chile rings, and a pinch of salt. Let the mixture sit for about 10 minutes, allowing the chile rings to soften a bit.
9. Add the capers and the remaining canola oil. Add salt and pepper to taste.
10. Drizzle chile vinaigrette over the roasted broccoli and salmon just before serving.

Salmon and Crispy Kale (With Coconut)

Ingredients:

- 1 cup coconut milk
- 1 cup uncooked jasmine rice, rinsed and drained well
- 1/3 cup coconut oil, melted
- 1/2 tsp. sea salt
- 1 cup water
- 2 tbsp. coconut aminos or tamari
- 1 tsp. sesame oil
- 1 tbsp. Sriracha
- 1 cup coconut flakes
- 1 bunch kale
- 1 lbs. salmon, cut into pieces

For the sweet potatoes:

- 3 sweet potatoes, yellow type, cubed
- 1 tbsp. coconut oil, melted
- 1 tsp. paprika

Instructions:
1. In a saucepan, add rice, coconut milk, water, and salt. Bring to a boil and stir.

5. Reduce heat and simmer for 15-20 minutes. Drain and rinse.
6. Place a steamer basket in a pot with water and bring to a boil.
7. Add broccoli. Cover and steam for 4-5 minutes then remove, keeping water in the pot.
8. Add squash. Cover and steam for 4-5 minutes then remove, keeping water in the pot.
9. Add chard. Cover and steam for 3-4 minutes, then remove.
10. Mix all the sauce ingredients in a small bowl. Set aside for serving later.
11. Plate everything as desired, with sauerkraut and sauce on the side or in a separate saucer.
12. Serve and enjoy!

Roasted Broccoli and Salmon

Ingredients;
- 1-1/2 lbs. or 1 bunch broccoli, cut into florets
- 4 tbsp. Canola oil, divided
- salt
- pepper
- 4 pcs. salmon fillets, deskinned
- 1 pc. jalapeño or red Fresno chile, deseeded and sliced into thin rings
- 2 tbsp. unseasoned rice vinegar
- 2 tbsp. capers, drained

Instructions:
1. Preheat the oven to 400° F.
2. Place broccoli florets in a large, rimmed baking sheet. Drizzle with 2 tbsp. canola oil and season with salt and pepper.
3. Roast the florets in the oven for 12 or 15 minutes. Toss occasionally.
4. Remove from the oven when the florets are crisp-tender and browned.
5. Gently rub the salmon fillets with 1 tbsp. of the canola oil. Season with salt and pepper.
6. Place the salmon in the middle of the baking sheet. Move the florets to the sides of the baking sheet.
7. Roast the fillet for 10 to 15 minutes or until the fillets turn opaque throughout.

8. Add the sausage mixture to the bowl with the rest of the ingredients.
9. Mix until everything is well blended.
10. Line the pan with some fat from the sausage or grease well with oil, butter, or ghee to prevent quiche from sticking.
11. Pour mixture into the cast iron pan or oven-safe dish.
12. Bake for 40-45 minutes or until a knife poked at the center comes out clean.
13. Serve and enjoy while warm.

Broccoli Soup with Tumeric and Ginger

Ingredients:

- 1 onion
- 3 cloves garlic
- 1 can unsweetened coconut milk
- 1 tsp. salt
- 1 tsp. turmeric powder
- 2 tsp. fresh ginger chopped
- 2 small heads of broccoli chopped into florets
- 1 cup of water
- Optional, for serving: fresh greens, roasted almonds, sesame seeds, and/or yogurt

Instructions:

1. In a pan over low heat, pour half of the coconut milk.
2. Add the garlic and onion. Cook until soft, for about 5 minutes.
3. Add the ginger, turmeric, florets, salt, water, and the rest of the coconut milk.
4. Simmer for an hour. Stir occasionally and mash the broccoli.
5. Allow the mixture to cool.
6. Blend the mixture in a food processor. Do in batches if needed.
7. Serve with a choice of sides or toppings.

Avocado Chicken Lemon Salad

Ingredients:
- 2 organic chicken breast, skinless
- a big bunch of curly kale, ribs and stems removed
- 1 cup of cooked wheat berries
- 1 ripe avocado, sliced and drizzled with lemon juice
- 1/2 cup pomegranate arils
- 1/2 cup toasted pine nuts
- pink peppercorns
- pea shoots

For the rosemary oil marinade:
- 1/2 lemon, zest only
- 1 sprig of rosemary
- 2 tbsp. olive oil
- sea salt
- black pepper

For the lemon vinaigrette:
- 1 tsp. dijon mustard
- 1-2 garlic cloves, minced
- 2 anchovy fillets, minced
- 2 tbsp. extra virgin olive oil
- 1 small lemon, juice only
- 1/2 tsp. lemon zest
- sea salt
- black pepper

Instructions:
1. Prepare the chicken by washing and draining with a paper towel.
2. Slice through the chicken breasts for the marinade and cook well later.
3. Using a mortar, mix all ingredients for the rosemary oil marinade until you get aromatic oil.
4. Gently rub the chicken with the rosemary oil and marinate for at least 15 minutes at room temperature or up to 8 hours in the refrigerator. Occasionally turn over the bag during the day.
5. Preheat the oven up to 375°F.
6. Heat cast-iron skillet over medium-high heat.
7. Add in chicken breasts. Cook until both sides are brown.
8. Move the skillet to the oven and cook for about 7-10 minutes.
9. Using a whisk, combine all the lemon vinaigrette ingredients in the bowl.
10. Put the kale and lemon vinaigrette in a large mixing bowl. Use your hands to mix for about a minute or two. Adjust seasoning according to your preference.
11. Move kale on a serving plate, topped with avocado slices.
12. Slice the chicken and place it on top of the salad. Top with peppercorns, pomegranate arils, toasted pine nuts, and wheat berries.
13. For garnishing, add pea shoots.

14. Enjoy by serving either warm or chilled, with the grilled lemon on the side.

Asparagus with Garlic and Onions

Ingredients

- 1/2 lb. fresh asparagus, trimmed
- 1/2 cup white onion, diced
- 3 tbsp. butter
- 1/4 cup water
- 2 cloves garlic, thinly sliced
- salt
- black pepper

Instructions:

1. Add water, asparagus, and onion into a skillet. Cover it.
2. Bring it to a boil over medium heat. Steam for about 2-5 minutes, or until the onion and asparagus are slightly tender.
3. If necessary, add a few tablespoons of water to maintain the steam.
4. After the water evaporates, add butter to the skillet.
5. Continue cooking until the asparagus and onions are lightly browned.
6. Throw in the garlic and cook for about half a minute more.
7. Add salt and pepper according to your taste.
8. Serve and enjoy while warm.

Mixed Vegetable Roast with Lemon Zest

Ingredients:
- 1-1/2 cups broccoli florets
- 1-1/2 cups cauliflower florets
- 3/4 cup red bell pepper, diced
- 3/4 cup zucchini, diced
- 2 thinly sliced cloves of garlic
- 2 tsp. lemon zest
- 1 tbsp. olive oil
- A pinch of salt
- 1 tsp. dried and crushed oregano

Instructions:
1. Preheat the oven at 425°F for 25 minutes.
2. Combine garlic and florets of broccoli and cauliflower in a baking pan.
3. Drizzle oil evenly over the vegetables. Season with salt and oregano.
4. Stir the vegetables to coat them evenly.
5. Place the pan inside the oven and roast for 10 minutes.
6. Add zucchini and bell pepper to the mix. Toss to combine.
7. Continue roasting for 10 to 15 minutes more until the vegetables turn light brown.
8. Drizzle lemon zest over vegetables and toss.
9. Serve and enjoy.

Conclusion

Thank you again for getting this guide.

If you found this guide helpful, please take the time to share your thoughts and post a review. It'd be greatly appreciated!

Thank   you   and   good   luck!

2. Reduce to the lowest heat. Cover and cook for 10 minutes. Remove from heat.
3. Preheat the oven to 390°F.
4. To make the dressing, add melted coconut oil, coconut aminos, sesame oil, and Sriracha in a lidded jar. Place the lid on the jar and shake vigorously until emulsified. Set aside.
5. On a baking sheet, put the sweet potatoes. Sprinkle melted coconut oil and paprika on top. Toss to coat.
6. Bake in the oven until tender or about half an hour.
7. On another baking sheet, add coconut flakes and kale.
8. Dress with about 2/3 of the dressing. Toss to coat well.
9. Drizzle 1-2 tbsp. of the dressing on the salmon.
10. Put the salmon and the coconut kale mixture in the oven, 15 minutes before the sweet potatoes' baking time, or until everything is cooked through.
11. Serve the salmon over fluffed rice with an extra drizzle of dressing. On a separate dish, place the sweet potatoes.

Green Salad

Ingredients:
- 5 cups mixed greens, such as romaine lettuce, arugula, swiss chard, mizuna, radicchio
- 1/4 red onion, sliced
- 2 tbsp. shelled sunflower seeds
- 1 medium-sized cucumber, thinly sliced
- 1/4 cup bacon bits

For the salad dressing:
- 1/4 cup honey
- 1/4 cup Dijon mustard
- 1/4 cup apple cider vinegar
- 1/4 cup virgin olive oil
- 1 tsp. salt

Instructions:
1. Put all the dressing ingredients in a covered jar. Shake vigorously to combine.
2. In a large salad bowl, combine all the mixed greens and other ingredients.
3. Serve   immediately.

Savory Chicken and Lentil Soup

Ingredients:

- 12 oz. or about 3 pcs. chicken thighs, remove bones, skin, and fat
- 1 lb. dried lentils
- 8 cups water
- 1/4 cup cilantro, chopped or minced
- 3 cloves garlic, minced
- 2 scallions, minced
- 1 ripe tomato, minced
- 1 onion, minced
- 1 tbsp. chicken stock
- 1 tsp. cumin
- 1 tsp. garlic powder
- 1/4 tsp. oregano
- 1/4 tsp. Spanish paprika, ground annatto seed, or Sazon seasoning
- Salt, to taste

Instructions:

1. Place chicken thighs, lentils, water, and chicken stock in a large pot.
2. Cover the pot before boiling using medium-low heat for about 20 minutes, or until the chicken thighs are cooked through.
3. Take out chicken thighs from the pot to shred them.
4. Return shredded chicken to the pot.
5. Add other ingredients, except salt, into the pot.

6. Boil for about 25 minutes, or until the lentils are cooked.
7. Pour more water if the soup has thickened too much.
8. Season with salt according to your taste.
9. Enjoy it while hot.

5. Pour the sauce over cooked quinoa. Garnish with pine nuts and basil leaves. Serve hot.

Spinach Quiche

Ingredients:
- 1 lb. breakfast sausage
- 1/2 onion, diced
- 2 cups mushrooms, sliced
- 6 cups spinach, roughly chopped
- 12 eggs
- 1/4 to 1/2 cup full-fat coconut milk
- 1 tsp. garlic powder
- 1 tsp. Italian seasoning
- 1 tsp. salt
- 1 tsp. pepper

Instructions:
1. Preheat the oven to 400°F.
2. Heat a cast-iron pan or another oven-safe pan over medium heat. Cook sausage and onion. Stir occasionally until sausage turns brown, about 7-8 minutes.
3. Add in mushrooms. Allow them to cook with the sausage until soft, for about 2 minutes. Remove from heat.
4. Crack eggs into a large bowl.
5. Add coconut milk. For a lighter and fluffier texture, use ½ cup. Use less for less coconut taste.
6. Whisk together well to get a light egg mixture.
7. Add spinach and seasonings to the bowl with the eggs.

Made in United States
Troutdale, OR
05/23/2024

20079845R20040